VEGANS WEIGHT GAIN COOKBOOK

:31 nutritious and flavorful meals to boost your calories intake

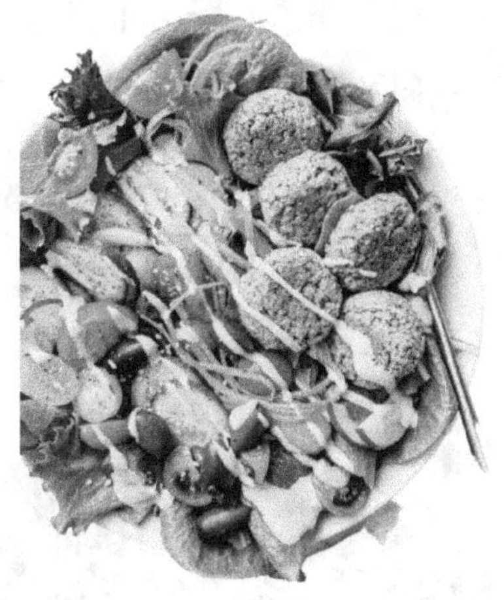

Dr. Malvin harison

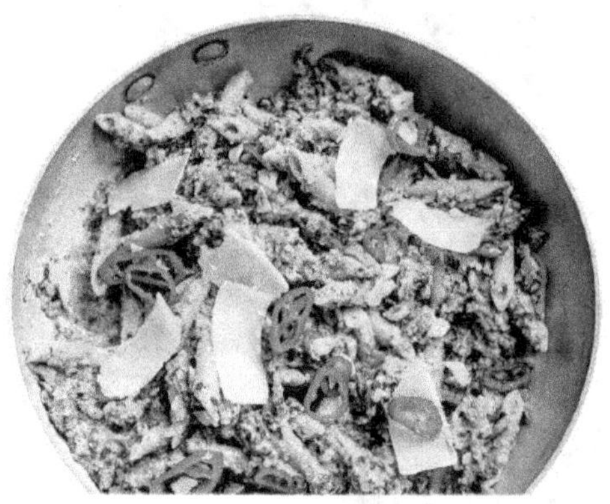

TABLE OF CONTENT

INTRODUCTION 3

10 BENEFITS OF GAINING WEIGHT ON VEGANS DIET..6

1.Improved Muscle Development: 6

2.Heart Health: 6

3.Digestive Health: 7

4.Lower Risk of Chronic Diseases: 7

5.Weight Management: 7

6.Increased Energy Levels: 8

7.Better Blood Sugar Control: 8

8.Enhanced Skin Health: 8

9. Positive Impact on the Environment: 8

10.Ethical and Compassionate Choice: 9

29 WEIGHT GAIN RECIPES FOR VEGANS WITH INSTRUCTIONS AND INGREDIENTS.................10

DELICIOUS BREAKFAST RECIPES: 10

1. High-Calorie Smoothie 10

2. Vegan Protein Pancakes 11

3. Coconut Chia Pudding 11

4. Peanut Butter Banana Toast......................12

5. Vegan Breakfast Burrito 12

6. Vegan French Toast 13

CRUNCHY LUNCH RECIPES FOR WEIGHT GAIN 14

7. Vegan Chickpea Tuna Salad 14

8. Veggie and Lentil Bowl 15

9. Vegan Eggplant Parmesan 17

10. Vegan Coconut Curry 19

11. Vegan Mushroom Stroganoff 19

12. Vegan Rice Pudding 20

13. Chickpea Avocado Salad 21

MOUTHWATERING DINNER RECIPES 22

16. Vegan Pasta 22

17. BBQ Jackfruit Sandwich 23

18. Vegan Stuffed Bell Peppers 23

19. Veggie Quinoa Bowl 24

20. Spicy Lentil Wraps 26

DELICIOUS HEALTHY SNACKS: 27

21. Trail Mix 27

22. Vegan Energy Bars 27

23. Hummus and Veggie Snack Plate 28

24. Vegan Chocolate Peanut Butter Shake 29

25. Vegan chocolate chips, melted 29

26. Caramelized Nuts 29

27. Vegan Avocado Chocolate Mousse 30

28. Vegan Spinach and Artichoke Dip 31

29. Vegan Banana Nut Muffins 31

DESSERTS: 33

30. Vegan Oatmeal Raisin Cookies 33

31. Vegan Chocolate Banana Bread 34

7-DAY MEAL PLAN FOR A VEGAN ON A WEIGHT GAIN DIET: **35**

DAY 1: 35

DAY 2: 35

DAY 3: 36

DAY 4: 36

DAY 5: 36

DAY 6: 36

DAY 7:...37
20 VEGANS SMOOTHIES FOR WEIGHT GAIN .37
1. Chocolate Peanut Butter Banana Shake 38
2. Tropical Mango Coconut Smoothie.............39
3. Peanut Butter and Jelly Smoothie...............39
4. Green Power Smoothie................................39
5. Strawberry Banana Nut Shake 40
6. Blueberry Almond Crunch Smoothie...........40
7. Cherry Vanilla Protein Shake......................40
8. Creamy Coconut Cashew Smoothie...........41
9. Mixed Berry Quinoa Smoothie 41
10. Mango Avocado Green Smoothie.............41
11. Chocolate Cherry Protein Shake 42
12. Pineapple Coconut Turmeric Smoothie 42
13. Berry Almond Butter Bliss Smoothie........42
14. Peaches and Cream Smoothie 43
15. Raspberry Coconut Chia Smoothie 43
16. Tropical Green Smoothie 43
17. Mango Macadamia Madness Smoothie....44
18. Blueberry Peanut Butter Power Smoothie 44
19. Pineapple Orange Creamsicle Smoothie..44
20. Vanilla Fig Pistachio Smoothie 45
CONCLUSION 46

INTRODUCTION

Welcome to the " Vegans Weight Gain Cookbook," a comprehensive guide designed to help you achieve your weight gain goals while following a nutritious and plant-based diet. Whether you are looking to increase muscle mass, gain healthy weight, or simply maintain a well-balanced lifestyle, this cookbook has you covered.

The vegan lifestyle has gained popularity over the years, and it offers numerous health benefits, including lower risks of heart disease, diabetes, and certain cancers. However, for some individuals, maintaining or gaining weight on a vegan diet can be a challenge. But fear not! This cookbook is here to show you that with the right ingredients, meal plans, and recipes, you can achieve your desired weight goals while enjoying delicious and satisfying vegan meals.

In this cookbook, you will find a diverse array of recipes thoughtfully crafted to provide the essential nutrients and calories needed for healthy weight gain. From hearty breakfast options and energizing lunches to hearty dinners and delectable snacks, each recipe has been designed to be both flavorful and calorie-dense.

Beyond just recipes, this cookbook also offers practical tips and nutritional insights to help you understand how to create balanced meals that promote weight gain and overall well-being. We'll explore the importance of macronutrients, portion control, and incorporating nutrient-dense foods to ensure you are getting the most out of your vegan weight gain journey.

So, whether you are a seasoned vegan looking to put on a few pounds or a newcomer to the plant-based lifestyle seeking guidance, this "Weight Gain Cookbook for Vegans" is your go-to resource. Get ready to embark on a delicious and fulfilling culinary adventure that will nourish both your body and soul.

10 BENEFITS OF GAINING WEIGHT ON VEGANS DIET

Gaining weight on a vegan diet can offer numerous benefits, as it allows individuals to achieve their weight goals while enjoying the advantages of a plant-based lifestyle. Here are ten benefits of gaining weight on a vegan diet:

1.Improved Muscle Development:

Gaining weight on a vegan diet can provide the necessary nutrients, such as plant-based protein, to support muscle growth and development, essential for athletes and fitness enthusiasts.

2.Heart Health:

A well-balanced vegan diet can be low in saturated fats and cholesterol, which can contribute to improved heart health and a reduced risk of cardiovascular diseases.

3.Digestive Health:

A vegan diet rich in whole grains, fruits, and vegetables provides dietary fiber, promoting healthy digestion and regular bowel movements.

4.Lower Risk of Chronic Diseases:

A vegan diet often includes an abundance of fruits and vegetables, which are high in antioxidants and phytochemicals. These compounds can help reduce inflammation and lower the risk of chronic diseases such as cancer and diabetes.

5.Weight Management:

Gaining weight in a controlled manner on a vegan diet can help individuals achieve and maintain a healthy weight, supporting overall well-being and reducing the risk of obesity-related health issues.

6.Increased Energy Levels:

Nutrient-dense vegan foods can provide a steady source of energy, making individuals feel more energized and alert throughout the day.

7.Better Blood Sugar Control:

A vegan diet can be beneficial for those with type 2 diabetes or those at risk of developing diabetes, as it may improve insulin sensitivity and glycemic control.

8.Enhanced Skin Health:

Plant-based foods rich in vitamins, minerals, and antioxidants can promote healthy skin, reducing the risk of skin issues and providing a natural glow.

9. Positive Impact on the Environment:

Gaining weight on a vegan diet contributes to a lower carbon footprint and reduced greenhouse gas emissions, as plant-based diets typically have a lower environmental impact compared to omnivorous diets.

10.Ethical and Compassionate Choice:

Embracing a vegan diet not only benefits personal health but also reflects a compassionate choice that advocates for the well-being of animals and supports sustainable agricultural practices.

29 WEIGHT GAIN RECIPES FOR VEGANS WITH INSTRUCTIONS AND INGREDIENTS

DELICIOUS BREAKFAST RECIPES:

1. High-Calorie Smoothie

Ingredients:

1 cup of coconut milk

1 ripe banana

1 tablespoon of almond butter

1 tablespoon of chia seeds

1 tablespoon of hemp seeds

1/2 cup of rolled oats

1 tablespoon of maple syrup

Instructions:

Blend all ingredients until smooth. Add more coconut milk if needed for desired consistency.

2. Vegan Protein Pancakes

Ingredients:

1 cup of whole wheat flour

1 tablespoon of baking powder

1 tablespoon of sugar

1 cup of almond milk

2 tablespoons of vegan protein powder

1 tablespoon of vegetable oil

Instructions:

In a bowl, mix the flour, baking powder, sugar, and protein powder.

Add almond milk and vegetable oil, and whisk until smooth.

Cook pancakes on a non-stick pan over medium heat until golden brown on each side.

3. Coconut Chia Pudding

Ingredients:

1/4 cup of chia seeds

1 cup of coconut milk

1 tablespoon of agave syrup

1/2 teaspoon of vanilla extract

Fresh berries for topping

Instructions:

Mix chia seeds, coconut milk, agave syrup, and vanilla extract in a jar.
Stir well and refrigerate overnight.
Serve with fresh berries on top.

4. Peanut Butter Banana Toast

Ingredients:
2 slices of whole-grain bread
2 tablespoons of peanut butter
1 ripe banana, cut into smaller pieces
1 tablespoon of chia seeds
1 tablespoon of maple syrup
Instructions:
Toast the bread slices until lightly browned.
Spread peanut butter on each slice.
Arrange sliced bananas on top.
Drizzle maple syrup and sprinkle chia seeds over the toast.

5. Vegan Breakfast Burrito

Ingredients:
4 large whole-grain tortillas
1 cup of firm tofu, crumbled
1 cup of black beans (cooked or canned)
1 cup of sliced bell peppers
1/2 cup of diced onions

1 teaspoon of turmeric powder
Salt and pepper to taste
Avocado slices and salsa for topping
Instructions:
In a skillet, sauté onions and bell peppers until softened.
Add crumbled tofu, black beans, turmeric, salt, and pepper. Cook for a few minutes.
Warm the tortillas and fill each with the tofu mixture.
Top with avocado slices and salsa before rolling them up.

6. Vegan French Toast

Ingredients:
4 slices of thick bread
1 cup of unsweetened almond milk
2 tablespoons of chickpea flour
1 tablespoon of nutritional yeast
1 teaspoon of vanilla extract
1/2 teaspoon of cinnamon
1 tablespoon of coconut oil for cooking
Fresh fruit and maple syrup for topping

Instructions:

In a shallow dish, whisk almond milk, chickpea flour, nutritional yeast, vanilla, and cinnamon.

Dip each slice of bread into the mixture, ensuring both sides are coated.

Heat the coconut oil in a non-stick pan over medium heat.

Cook each slice of bread until golden brown on both sides.

Serve with fresh fruit and drizzle with maple syrup.

CRUNCHY LUNCH RECIPES FOR WEIGHT GAIN

7. Vegan Chickpea Tuna Salad

Ingredients:
1 can of chickpeas (drained and rinsed)
1/4 cup of vegan mayonnaise
1 tablespoon of dijon mustard
2 tablespoons of lemon juice
1/4 cup of diced celery
1/4 cup of diced red onion
2 tablespoons of chopped dill
Salt and pepper to taste
Lettuce leaves for serving
Instructions:

In a bowl, mash the chickpeas with a fork or potato masher.

Add vegan mayonnaise, dijon mustard, lemon juice, celery, red onion, dill, salt, and pepper. Mix well.

Serve on lettuce leaves as a salad or use it to make sandwiches.

8. Veggie and Lentil Bowl

Ingredients:

1 cup of cooked brown rice

1 cup of cooked green lentils

1 cup of sautéed spinach

1/2 cup of roasted cherry tomatoes

1/4 cup of sliced avocado

2 tablespoons of balsamic vinaigrette

Instructions:

Arrange rice, lentils, spinach, cherry tomatoes, and avocado in a bowl.

Drizzle with balsamic vinaigrette.

9. Vegan Eggplant Parmesan

Ingredients:

1 large eggplant, sliced into rounds

1 cup of breadcrumbs (use panko for extra crispiness)

1 cup of marinara sauce

1 cup of vegan mozzarella cheese

1/4 cup of nutritional yeast

Fresh basil leaves for garnish

Olive oil for baking

Instructions:

Preheat the oven to 375°F (190°C).

Dip eggplant slices in marinara sauce, then coat them with breadcrumbs mixed with nutritional yeast.

Lay the coated eggplant slices on a baking sheet lined with parchment paper.

Bake for 20 minutes, flipping halfway through, until crispy and golden.

Top with vegan mozzarella cheese and bake for an additional 5-7 minutes or until cheese melts.

Garnish with fresh basil leaves before serving.

10. Vegan Coconut Curry

Ingredients:

1 cup of cooked chickpeas

1 cup of diced sweet potatoes

1 cup of chopped cauliflower

1 cup of sliced bell peppers

1 can of coconut milk

2 tablespoons of red curry paste

1 tablespoon of soy sauce

1 tablespoon of lime juice

Fresh cilantro for garnish

Instructions:

In a large pot, simmer chickpeas, sweet potatoes, cauliflower, and bell peppers in coconut milk and red curry paste.

Add soy sauce and lime juice, and cook until vegetables are tender.

Garnish with fresh cilantro before serving over rice or quinoa.

11. Vegan Mushroom Stroganoff

Ingredients:

8 ounces of vegan egg noodles (cooked according to package instructions)

2 cups of sliced mushrooms

1 cup of chopped onions

1 cup of vegetable broth

1 cup of cashew cream (blend 1 cup soaked cashews with 1 cup water until smooth)

2 tablespoons of soy sauce

1 tablespoon of Dijon mustard

2 cloves of garlic, minced

Salt and pepper to taste

Fresh parsley for garnish

Instructions:

In a large skillet, make the mushrooms and onions tender.

Add vegetable broth, cashew cream, soy sauce, Dijon mustard, garlic, salt, and pepper.

Cook until the sauce thickens.

Serve with cooked egg, noodles and garnish with fresh parsley.

12. Vegan Rice Pudding

Ingredients:

1 cup of cooked white rice

1 can of coconut milk

1/4 cup of maple syrup

1 teaspoon of vanilla extract

1/2 teaspoon of cinnamon

1/4 cup of raisins

Instructions:

In a saucepan, combine cooked rice, coconut milk, maple syrup, vanilla extract, and cinnamon.
Cook with medium heat, stir it frequently, until the mixture becomes thick.
Add raisins and cook for an additional 2-3 minutes.
Serve warm or chilled.

13. Chickpea Avocado Salad

Ingredients:
1 can of chickpeas (drained and rinsed)
1 ripe avocado (sliced)
1/2 cup of cherry tomatoes (halved)
1/4 cup of diced cucumber
2 tablespoons of lemon juice
Salt and pepper to taste
Instructions:
In a bowl, combine chickpeas, avocado, cherry tomatoes, and cucumber.
Splash lemon juice over the salad and add salt and pepper to taste. Toss gently.

MOUTHWATERING DINNER RECIPES

16. Vegan Pasta

Ingredients:

8 ounces of fettuccine (cooked according to package instructions)

1 cup of whole cashews (soaked in water for 2 hours)

1 cup of vegetable broth

2 tablespoons of nutritional yeast

2 small garlic cloves

Juice from 1 lemon

Salt and pepper to taste

Fresh parsley for garnish

Instructions:

In a blender, blend soaked cashews, vegetable broth, nutritional yeast, garlic, and lemon juice until smooth.

Pour the sauce over cooked fettuccine and toss to coat.

Season with salt and pepper and garnish with fresh parsley.

17. BBQ Jackfruit Sandwich

Ingredients:

1 can of amateur green jackfruit (drained and shredded)

1/2 cup of barbecue sauce

4 burger buns

Sliced pickles and coleslaw for topping

Instructions:

Heat shredded jackfruit in a pan and add barbecue sauce. Cook until heated through.

Toast burger buns and fill them with the jackfruit mixture.

Top with pickles and coleslaw.

18.Vegan Stuffed Bell Peppers

Ingredients:

4 bell peppers (any color)

1 cup of cooked quinoa

1 cup of black beans (cooked or canned)

1 cup of sliced tomatoes

1/2 cup of corn kernels

1 teaspoon cumin

1 teaspoon paprika

Salt and pepper to taste

Instructions:

Preheat the oven to 375°F (190°C).

Remove the tops of the bell peppers and remove seeds.

In a bowl, mix quinoa, black beans, diced tomatoes, corn, cumin, paprika, salt, and pepper.

Add each bell pepper with the quinoa mixture and place them in a baking dish.

Bake until the peppers are tender.

19. Veggie Quinoa Bowl

Ingredients:

1 cup of cooked quinoa

1 cup of steamed broccoli florets

1/2 cup of roasted sweet potatoes (cubed)

1/4 cup of sliced almonds

2 tablespoons of tahini dressing

Instructions:

Arrange quinoa, broccoli, and sweet potatoes in a bowl.

Sprinkle sliced almonds on top and drizzle with tahini dressing.

20. Spicy Lentil Wraps

Ingredients:

1 cup of cooked lentils

1/4 cup of diced bell peppers

1/4 cup of shredded carrots

1/4 cup of chopped red onions

2 tablespoons of hot sauce

4 whole-grain tortillas

Instructions:

Mix cooked lentils, bell peppers, carrots, and red onions in a bowl.

Add hot sauce and stir until well combined.

Divide the lentil mixture into tortillas and roll them into wAlfredoraps.

DELICIOUS HEALTHY SNACKS:

21. Trail Mix

Ingredients:
1 cup of mixed nuts (almonds, cashews, walnuts)
½ cup of pumpkin seeds
1/2 cup of dried cranberries
1/4 cup of dark chocolate chips
Instructions:
Combine all ingredients in a bowl and store in a tight container.

22. Vegan Energy Bars

Ingredients:
1 cup of dates (pitted)
1 cup of rolled oats
1/2 cup of almond butter
1/4 cup of maple syrup
1/4 cup of shredded coconut
1/4 cup of vegan chocolate chips
Instructions:
Blend dates in a food processor until a sticky paste forms.

Add oats, almond butter, maple syrup, and shredded coconut. Pulse until combined.

Transfer the mixture to a lined baking dish and press it down firmly.

Sprinkle chocolate chips on top and refrigerate for 1-2 hours before cutting into bars.

23. Hummus and Veggie Snack Plate

Ingredients:

1 cup of hummus

Sliced cucumber, carrots, and bell peppers

Whole wheat pita bread or crackers

Instructions:

Arrange hummus and sliced vegetables on a plate.

Serve with whole wheat pita bread or crackers for dipping.

Feel free to modify and adjust the recipes according to your taste preferences and dietary needs.

24. Vegan Chocolate Peanut Butter Shake

Ingredients:

1 cup of unsweetened almond milk

2 tablespoons of cocoa powder

2 tablespoons of peanut butter

1 ripe banana

1 teaspoon of maple syrup (optional, for added sweetness)

Instructions:

Blend all ingredients until well combined and frothy.

25. Vegan chocolate chips, melted

26. Caramelized Nuts

Ingredients:

1 cup of mixed nuts (almonds, cashews, and walnuts)

1/4 cup of maple syrup

1/2 teaspoon of cinnamon

Pinch of salt

Instructions

In a pan, heat maple syrup, cinnamon, and salt. Add the mixed nuts and stir until they are well coated and caramelized. Spread them out on a parchment-lined baking sheet and let them cool.

27. Vegan Avocado Chocolate Mousse

Ingredients:
2 ripe avocados
1/4 cup of cocoa powder
1/4 cup of maple syrup
1 teaspoon of vanilla extract
Pinch of salt
Fresh berries for topping
Instructions:
In a blender or food processor, blend avocados, cocoa powder, maple syrup, vanilla extract, and salt until smooth and creamy.
Place in the refrigerator and let it chill for at least 1 hour before serving.
Top with fresh berries.

28. Vegan Spinach and Artichoke Dip

Ingredients:

2 cups of fresh spinach leaves

A can of artichoke hearts (drained and chopped)

1 cup of vegan cream cheese

1/2 cup of vegan mayonnaise

1/4 cup of nutritional yeast

2 cloves of garlic, minced

Salt and pepper to taste

Tortilla chips or veggie sticks for dipping

Instructions:

In a saucepan, sauté spinach and chopped artichoke hearts until wilted.

Add vegan cream cheese, vegan mayonnaise, nutritional yeast, minced garlic, salt, and pepper. Mix until well combined and heat it thoroughly.

Dish with tortilla chips or veggie sticks for dipping.

29. Vegan Banana Nut Muffins

Ingredients:

2 ripe bananas, mashed

1/4 cup of coconut oil, melted

1/2 cup of maple syrup

1/2 cup of unsweetened almond milk

2 cups of all-purpose flour

1 teaspoon of baking powder

1/2 teaspoon of baking soda

1/2 teaspoon of cinnamon

1/4 teaspoon salt

1/2 cup of chopped walnuts

Instructions:

Preheat the oven to 350°F (175°C) and line a muffin tin with paper liners.

In a bowl, mix mashed bananas, coconut oil, maple syrup, and almond milk.

In a separate bowl, whisk together flour, baking powder, baking soda, cinnamon, and salt.

Combine wet and dry ingredients and fold in chopped walnuts.

Fill each muffin cup with batter and bake until a toothpick inserted in the center comes out clean.

DESSERTS:

30. Vegan Oatmeal Raisin Cookies

Ingredients:

1 and 1/2 cups of rolled oats

1 cup of all-purpose flour

1 teaspoon of baking soda

1/2 teaspoon of cinnamon

1/4 teaspoon of salt

1/2 cup of coconut oil, melted

1/2 cup of maple syrup

1 teaspoon of vanilla extract

1/2 cup of raisins

Instructions:

Preheat the oven to 350°F (175°C) and line a baking sheet with parchment paper.

In a bowl, mix rolled oats, flour, baking soda, cinnamon, and salt.

In another bowl, whisk together melted coconut oil, maple syrup, and vanilla extract.

Combine wet and dry ingredients and fold in raisins.

Form dough into cookies and place them on the baking sheet.

Bake for 12-15 minutes or until the edges turn golden brown.

31. Vegan Chocolate Banana Bread

Ingredients:

3 ripe bananas, mashed

1/2 cup of unsweetened applesauce

1/4 cup of coconut oil, melted

1/2 cup of maple syrup

1 teaspoon of vanilla extract

1 and 1/2 cups of all-purpose flour

1/2 cup of cocoa powder

1 teaspoon of baking powder

1/2 teaspoon of baking soda

1/4 teaspoon of salt

1/2 cup of vegan chocolate chips

Instructions:

Preheat the oven to 350°F (175°C) and grease a loaf pan.

In a bowl, mix mashed bananas, applesauce, melted coconut oil, maple syrup, and vanilla extract.

In another bowl, whisk together flour, cocoa powder, baking powder, baking soda, and salt.

Combine wet and dry ingredients and fold in vegan chocolate chips.

Pour the batter into the greased loaf pan and smooth the top.

Bake for 50-60 minutes or until a toothpick inserted in the center comes out clean.

7-DAY MEAL PLAN FOR A VEGAN ON A WEIGHT GAIN DIET:

DAY 1:

Breakfast: High-Calorie Smoothie
Lunch: Vegan Chickpea Tuna Salad
Dinner: Vegan Coconut Curry

DAY 2:

Breakfast: Vegan Protein Pancakes
Lunch: Veggie and Lentil Bowl
Dinner: Vegan Mushroom Stroganoff

DAY 3:

Breakfast: Vegan Oatmeal Raisin Cookies (as a treat)
Lunch: BBQ Jackfruit Sandwich
Dinner: Vegan Eggplant Parmesan

DAY 4:

Breakfast: Vegan Chocolate Banana Bread (as a treat)
Lunch: Spicy Lentil Wraps
Dinner: Vegan Stuffed Bell Peppers

DAY 5:

Breakfast: Vegan French Toast (as a treat)
Lunch: Vegan Avocado Chocolate Mousse (as a treat)
Dinner: Vegan Alfredo Pasta

DAY 6:

Breakfast: Peanut Butter Banana Toast
Lunch: Chickpea Avocado Salad
Dinner: Vegan Lentil Shepherd's Pie

DAY 7:

Breakfast: Coconut Chia Pudding
Lunch: Vegan Cheese and Crackers (as a snack)
Dinner: Vegan Lentil Loaf

20 VEGANS SMOOTHIES FOR WEIGHT GAIN

20 vegan smoothie recipes designed to support weight gain while providing essential nutrients and delicious flavors:

Here's one set of instructions that can be used for all the smoothie recipes:

Instructions:
Add all the ingredients listed for the chosen smoothie recipe into a high-speed blender.

Blend on high until smooth and creamy. If the mixture is too thick, you can add a little more liquid (e.g., almond milk, coconut water) to achieve your desired consistency.

Then, you can pour the smoothie into a cup and enjoy it immediately.

Optional: For added texture and presentation, you can top your smoothie with extra fruit, nuts, seeds, or a sprinkle of cocoa powder.

1. Chocolate Peanut Butter Banana Shake

1 cup of almond milk
1 ripe banana
2 tablespoons of peanut butter
1 tablespoon of cocoa powder
1 tablespoon of chia seeds
1 tablespoon of maple syrup

2. Tropical Mango Coconut Smoothie

1 cup of coconut milk
1 cup of frozen mango chunks
1/2 ripe avocado
1 tablespoon of hemp seeds
1 tablespoon of agave syrup

3. Peanut Butter and Jelly Smoothie

1 cup of oat milk
1/2 cup if frozen mixed berries
2 tablespoons of peanut butter
1 tablespoon of chia seeds
1 tablespoon of jam (your favorite flavor)

4. Green Power Smoothie

1 cup of spinach
1 ripe banana
1/2 cup of pineapple chunks
1 tablespoon of almond butter
1 tablespoon of flaxseed meal
1 cup of coconut water

5. Strawberry Banana Nut Shake

1 cup of almond milk
1 cup of frozen strawberries
1 ripe banana
1/4 cup of walnuts
1 tablespoon of maple syrup

6. Blueberry Almond Crunch Smoothie

1 cup of almond milk
1/2 cup of frozen blueberries
1/4 cup of rolled oats
2 tablespoons of almond butter
1 tablespoon of agave syrup

7. Cherry Vanilla Protein Shake

1 cup of soy milk
1 cup of frozen cherries
1/2 teaspoon of vanilla extract
1 tablespoon of hemp seeds
1 scoop of vegan vanilla protein powder

8. Creamy Coconut Cashew Smoothie

1 cup of coconut milk
1/4 cup of cashews
1 ripe banana
1 tablespoon of coconut oil
1 tablespoon of maple syrup

9. Mixed Berry Quinoa Smoothie

1 cup of almond milk
1/2 cup of mixed berries (strawberries, raspberries, blackberries)
1/4 cup of cooked quinoa
1 tablespoon of almond butter
1 tablespoon of agave syrup

10. Mango Avocado Green Smoothie

1 cup of coconut water
1 cup of fresh spinach
1/2 ripe of avocado
1 cup of frozen mango chunks
1 tablespoon of chia seeds
1 tablespoon of agave syrup

11. Chocolate Cherry Protein Shake

1 cup of almond milk
1 cup of frozen cherries
2 tablespoons of cocoa powder
1 tablespoon of almond butter
1 scoop of vegan chocolate protein powder

12. Pineapple Coconut Turmeric Smoothie

1 cup of coconut milk
1 cup of frozen pineapple chunks
1/2 ripe banana
1/2 teaspoon of turmeric powder
1 tablespoon of maple syrup

13. Berry Almond Butter Bliss Smoothie

1 cup of almond milk
1 cup of berries (it can be strawberries, blueberries, or raspberries)
2 tablespoons of almond butter
1 tablespoon of flaxseed meal
1 tablespoon of agave syrup

14. Peaches and Cream Smoothie

1 cup of soy milk
1 cup of frozen peaches
1/4 cup of rolled oats
1 tablespoon of almond butter
1 tablespoon of agave syrup

15. Raspberry Coconut Chia Smoothie

1 cup of coconut milk
1 cup of frozen raspberries
1 tablespoon of chia seeds
1 tablespoon of almond butter
1 tablespoon of maple syrup

16. Tropical Green Smoothie

1 cup of coconut water
1 cup of fresh spinach
1/2 cup of frozen pineapple chunks
1/2 ripe banana
1 tablespoon of hemp seeds
1 tablespoon of agave syrup

17. Mango Macadamia Madness Smoothie

1 cup of almond milk
1 cup of frozen mango chunks
1/4 cup of macadamia nuts
1 tablespoon of coconut oil
1 tablespoon of agave syrup

18. Blueberry Peanut Butter Power Smoothie

1 cup of soy milk
1/2 cup of frozen blueberries
2 tablespoons of peanut butter
1 tablespoon of chia seeds
1 tablespoon of agave syrup

19. Pineapple Orange Creamsicle Smoothie

1 cup of orange juice
1 cup of frozen pineapple chunks
1/2 ripe banana
1/4 cup of cashews
1 tablespoon of maple syrup

20. Vanilla Fig Pistachio Smoothie

1 cup of almond milk
2 ripe figs
1/4 cup of shelled pistachios
1 tablespoon of agave syrup
1/2 teaspoon of vanilla extract

CONCLUSION

Congratulations! You've reached the end of the "Vegans Weight Gain Cookbook." We hope that this culinary journey has not only provided you with scrumptious and nutrient-packed recipes but also encourages you to acquire a healthier and more fulfilling lifestyle.

Remember, weight gain on a vegan diet doesn't mean sacrificing flavor or variety. With the right knowledge and creativity, you can transform ordinary plant-based ingredients into delightful, calorie-rich meals that support your weight goals and nurture your well-being.

As you continue your vegan weight gain journey, don't forget the power of balance and consistency. Embrace a varied diet that includes a wide range of whole foods, fresh produce, legumes, nuts, and seeds. Experiment with different recipes, listen to your body's signals, and make adjustments as needed.

Whether you're seeking to build muscle, boost your energy, or simply feel more confident in your body, know that the choices you make in

the kitchen play a significant role in shaping
your overall health and happiness. As you
continue to enjoy the benefits of a vegan
lifestyle, always remember that nourishing
yourself with love and compassion is the
ultimate recipe for a fulfilling and joyful life.

Enjoy your vegan weight gain journey!

Happy cooking and bon appétit!

www.ingramcontent.com/pod-product-compliance
Lightning Source LLC
Chambersburg PA
CBHW070744260726
48660CB00007B/2969